Hatha YOGA

*The Ultimate Beginner's Guide
to Discover Yoga, Its History, and Philosophy*

Shreyanada Natha

Cover & design
Mattias Långström

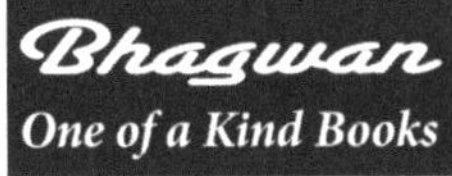

YOGA BEYOND THE POSES

Hatha YOGA

*The Ultimate Beginner's Guide
to Discover Yoga, Its History, and Philosophy*

Shreyanada Natha

ISBN 9789198839203

✳ ✳ ✳

2 FREE PREMIUM BONUS!

#1. *Download the* **AUDIOBOOK** *at the back of the book!*

#2. *Download* **CHAKRA-INDEX IN COLOR** *here!*

SCAN QR-CODE or go to:

https://bit.ly/47wdFVZ

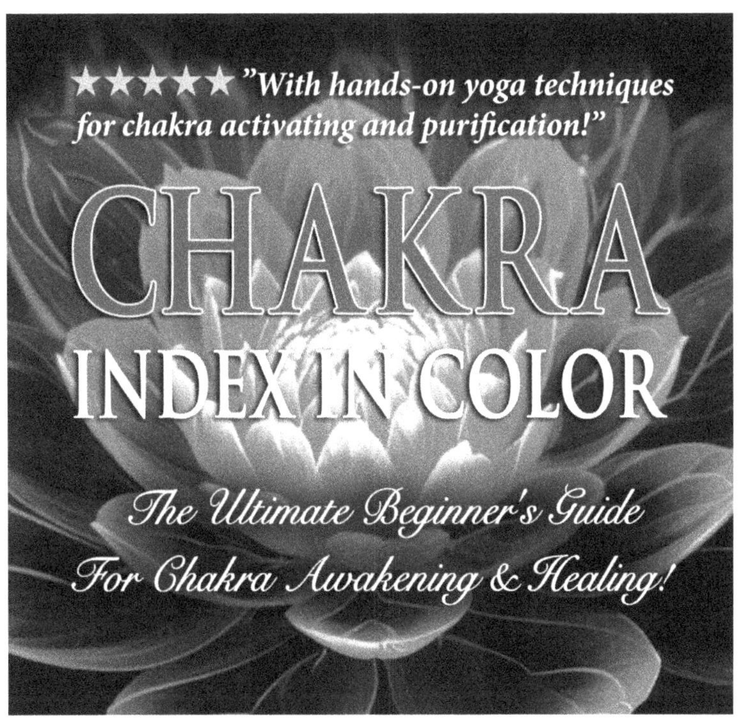

FREE PREMIUM Audiobook
Authentic Yoga Nidra Meditation – Ajna Chakra Awakening!

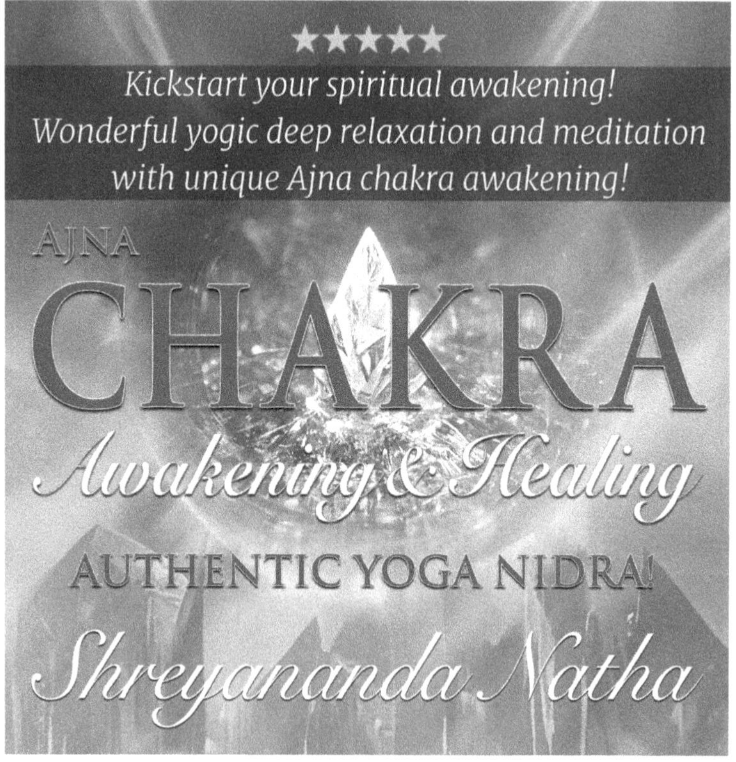

*Download the **AUDIOBOOK** at the back of the book!*

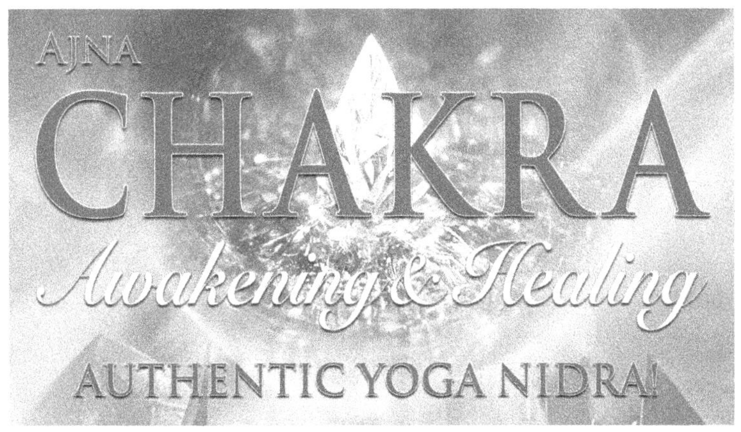

Kickstart your spiritual awakening! Wonderful yogic deep relaxation and meditation with unique Ajna chakra awakening and healing.

PRESENTATION

Yoga Nidra, or yogic sleep, is a unique meditation process that's powerfully profound and healing for body, mind, and spirit.

Practitioners are led into a state of deep relaxation and the experience of our chakra system.

Yoga Nidra offers extensive benefits, yet it is one of the most straightforward yoga practices.

All you have to do is put on your most comfortable clothes, find a quiet space, lie down on your back, and play the meditation.

Yoga Beyond the Poses – Hatha Yoga
The Ultimate Beginner's Guide to Discover Yoga, Its History, and Philosophy!
Including A Premium Audiobook: Yoga Nidra Meditation – Ajna Chakra Awakening And Healing!

The history behind yin yoga and modern yoga: Hatha yoga, asanas, pranayamas, mudras, bandhas, yoga history, and yoga philosophy.

The book "Hatha Yoga – My Body is My Temple" describes Hatha yoga, its origins, and mystique from the ground up. It delves deep but remains easily readable, educational, and straightforward—a must-have on the bookshelf for anyone interested in Hatha yoga and who wants to learn more quickly. The book is part of a series of seven yoga books, Yoga Beyond the Poses: The Ultimate Beginner's Guide to Yoga, that delve into the seven key areas of yoga.

INCLUDING A PREMIUM AUDIOBOOK: AUTHENTIC YOGA NIDRA MEDITATION – AJNA CHAKRA AWAKENING & HEALING!
Kickstart your spiritual awakening! Wonderful yogic deep relaxation and meditation with unique Ajna chakra awakening and healing.

Yoga Nidra, or yogic sleep, is a unique meditation process

that`s powerfully profound and healing for body, mind, and spirit. Practitioners are led into a state of deep relaxation and the experience of our chakra system. Yoga Nidra offers extensive benefits, yet it is one of the most straightforward yoga practices. All you have to do is put on your most comfortable clothes, find a quiet space, lie down on your back, and play the meditation. –
Download the audiobook at the back of the book!

ABOUT THE BOOK SERIES
YOGA BEYOND THE POSES: *The Ultimate Beginner's Guide to Yoga!*

The book is part of a seven-book yoga series, Yoga Beyond the Poses: The Ultimate Beginner's Guide to Yoga, that delve into yoga's seven most important areas. They are straightforward to read, educational, and fascinating. A must on the bookshelf for anyone interested in yoga who quickly wants to know more.

MY NAME AND MY MISSION

Shreyananda Natha was the name I was given when I was initiated into the Natha Order and received the master mantra – the Shodasi mantra, after studying yoga and tantra for over twelve years, the highest mantra in yoga and tantra. It means "he who knows".

After practicing yoga and meditation continuously for over twenty years, having a yoga school for many years, and leading studies for yoga teachers, I wanted to get out more widely with yoga into our whole society, out of the small yoga room. Spread the knowledge of yoga, our chakra system, and Kundalini Shakti to anyone who will listen. What needed to be added were educational fact books on yoga that didn't just skim the surface or deal with the author's private life. So it became my Sankalpa, my magical wish, and my mission to create exciting yoga books that everyone should be able to read and enjoy. To show how we can apply and use yoga in different areas of life and achieve success and health. Here and now.

If you like my books, feel free to follow me on my social media, share and like, tell your friends about the books, and write an honest review; one or two lines don't matter. All support is precious.

Thanks!

THE AUTHOR

Shreyananda Natha is the author of popular and best-selling yoga books. He has, among other things, written one of the most comprehensive books about yoga – EVERYTHING ABOUT YOGA and the study book – TEACHING YOGA AND MEDITATION BEYOND THE POSES. He is also a certified yoga and meditation teacher according to the EYTF international guidelines. He has undergone multi-year yoga teacher training under the guidance of Swami Omananda at Satyananda Ashram and holds the highest initiation in the tantric Natha order. He frequently travels to Asia and India to learn and gain knowledge and inspiration. He has immersed himself in tantric rituals and is known for his extensive knowledge of yoga, deep relaxation, and meditation.

"There is no authority that can say what yoga is. When you surrender yourself completely and fully and experience yoga without limitations and doubts, the true encounter with yoga occurs when you become one with the true experience within you. Only then will you understand what yoga is – for you. When you are no longer limited by neatness, shyness, and artificial thought patterns that act as a filter between you and the transformation. Yoga is a cultural-historical wealth still passed on from teacher to student and helps man find his way back to his true nature. It opens us up and attracts awareness. It strengthens our self-esteem, and our person's entire spectrum of possibilities suddenly becomes visible.

Yoga is not difficult or strange. You don't have to become a vegan, a monk, or be able to stand on your head. You just need to do your yoga regularly; the rest will take care of itself. You can use yoga and meditation to feel better, both physically and mentally, but also to achieve success and develop in all areas of life – here and now."

Good luck!

Namasté

I want to thank the teachers and students I've had over the years who have made my journey with yoga so enjoyable. Thank you for all the inspiration you have given me and for making this book possible. The yoga masters who no longer live among us – live on with each new person who immerses themselves in the yoga tradition.

Sri Swami Sivananda, Sri Swami Satyananda, Sri Tirumalai Krishnamacharya, Sri Swami Vishnudevananda, Sri K. Pattabhi Jois, Osho, Swami Nirdosha, Swami Omananda, Swami Janakananda, Ole Schmidt, Turiya, Maryam Abrishami and Sanna Kuittinen.

People who all searched for answers to what they sensed through an activated Ajna chakra. In yoga, they have learned the principles behind the universe, the collective consciousness, and the creative force, Kundalini Shakti. The duality behind everything, both what we see and what we don't see. Together, we are helped to pass on the previously secret knowledge about our gunas, nadis, and chakras to all who want to become a Rishi.

Aum Shri Durgayai Namaha

Shreyananda Natha

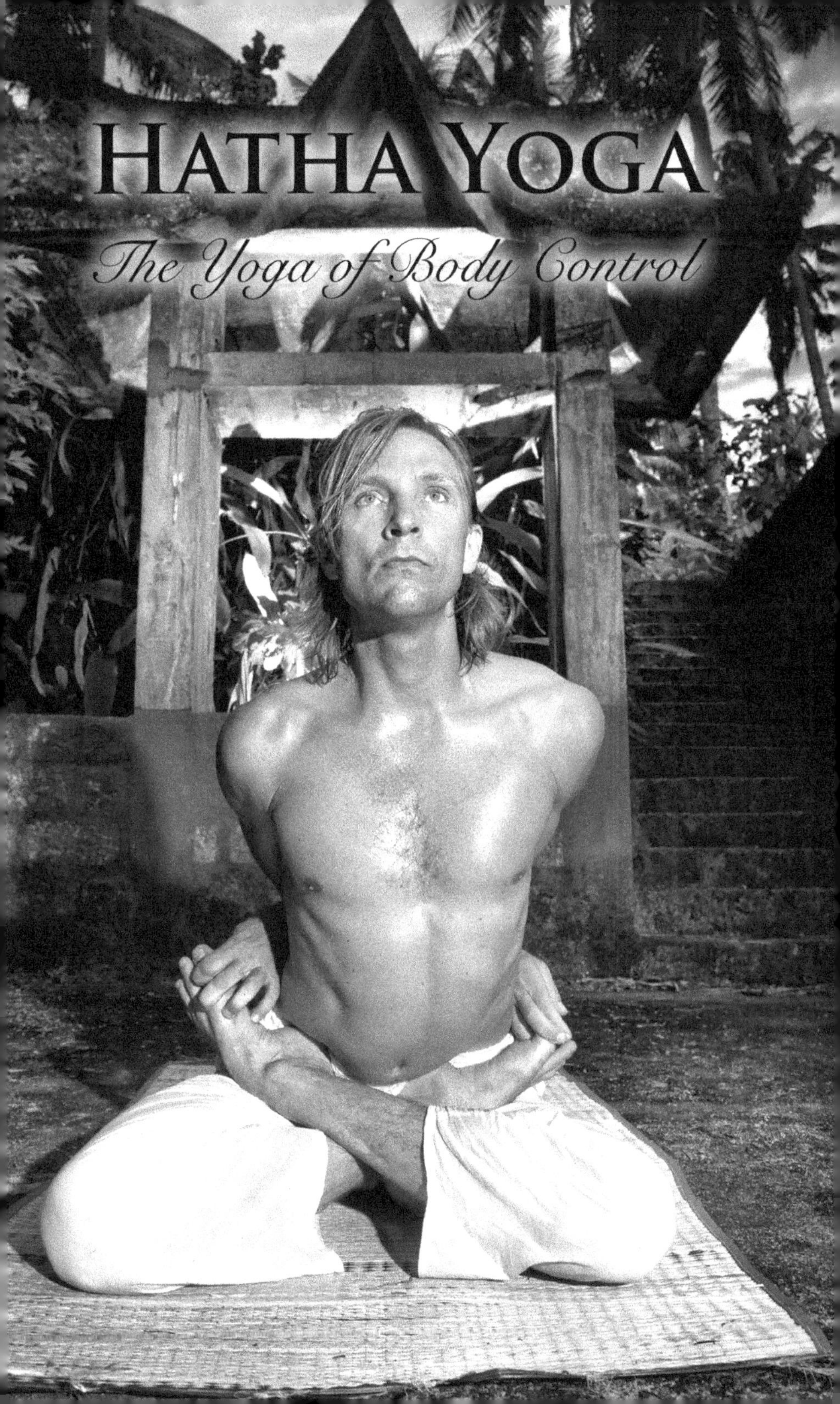

HATHA YOGA
The Yoga of Body Control

WHAT IS YOGA?

DEFINITION OF YOGA

Yoga chitta vritti nirodha (Yoga Sutras 1.2).
When the mind stills, yoga occurs.

THE MEANING OF YOGA

Yoga means unity and is derived from the word – yuj, which means to unite in Sanskrit. This unity or connection in the spiritual sense aims to connect individual consciousness with universal consciousness. In practice, this aims to balance and find harmony between body, mind, and emotions—a link between body and soul.

THE PURPOSE OF YOGA

He who knows Kundalini knows yoga. The Kundalini, it's said, is coiled like a serpent. He who can induce her to move is liberated (Hatha Yoga Pradipika v.105-111).

The absolute purpose of yoga is to awaken Kundalini Shakti and make her flow; this is a precondition for human evolution. Kundalini Shakti flows in the sushumna nadi along the spine and activates our most important chakras. They are in contact with the brain's untapped resources. When they are used, latent forces are released, and we are initiated into the universe's secrets. We become enlightened and get paranormal abilities – siddhis.

THE GOAL OF YOGA

We can define yoga from a classical perspective, its purpose and meaning, but there is no authority to prescribe the goal of yoga for you. Do you want to reach spiritual goals, get help to rid yourself of back problems, or perhaps just be free from demands and stress a few minutes a week?

There is undoubtedly a big difference in the stated goal of yoga if you practice with Aghori sadhus or among orthodox Hindu swamis. Even more significant is the difference between Chinese yoga practitioners and atheists in the Americanized Ashtanga industry. It is and has always been this way; this is the divine essence of yoga. It is as accessible and amorphous in purpose as in the feeling inside us. Yoga is indeed an infinite toolbox. Free to use for what matters most to us. Anandamaya kosha – yoga is unmanifested as our innermost self. When we experience all the power in the universe and on earth – inside and around – we decide for ourselves what the goal of yoga is for us.

THE ORIGIN OF YOGA

The yoga we know today has evolved as part of the Tantric civilization. Some believe the first yogi lived about five thousand years BCE; others believe that yoga is far older than that.

What we do know is that in the Indus Valley in Harappa and Mohenjodaro (Pakistan), where the pre-Vedic people once lived around 2600 BCE, statues depicting Shiva and Shakti (Parvati) have been found through archaeological excavations.

According to the myth, Shiva is the founder of yoga, and Parvati is his first disciple. Shiva is seen as a symbol (embodiment) of the highest consciousness. Parvati is considered the mother of the universe. She is the creator and represents knowledge, will, and action. This power, characterized as Kundalini Shakti, is dormant in every human being. Parvati conveyed the secret wisdom of human liberation through tantra, where yoga has its roots and cannot be separated, just as consciousness (Shiva) cannot be separated from energy (Shakti).

Yoga originated during the beginning of human civilization. Humans began to discover man's spiritual potential and developed techniques to develop it further. In the past, yoga was kept secret; it was not written down or performed publicly. Yoga was passed on orally from guru to student.

Tantric books are the first to refer to yoga and later to the Vedic scriptures. Rigveda, the oldest Vedic work, was written in 3-5000 BCE, probably by the Indus-Saraswati people. They are a collection of hymns written during a time when the culture in the Indus Valley was flourishing.

According to legend, Shiva (pure consciousness) taught Parvati (Shakti) yoga. A fish overheard their conversation, and Shiva turned the fish into a human. Not only animals would have yoga, but also humans.

VEDIC YOGA / ARCHAIC YOGA

Dating back to 5000 BCE, Vedic yoga is the oldest form. Sacrifice was seen as a path to the union between inner life, the sensual, and outer life, the material. To practice certain rituals and religions based on the Vedic hymns (which can be compared to the Old Testament), one had to focus and concentrate for an extended period, and to achieve this, yogic techniques were developed. Today, this remains the basis of yoga: to use inner focus to increase sensory and human abilities.

Vedic yoga was passed on by rishis (seers), not from guru to student.

PRE-CLASSICAL YOGA

The Upanishads form part of the Vedic scriptures, considered an essential work between 2000 BCE and 200 CE. The Upanishads consist of two hundred Gnostic texts in which yoga is mentioned. Yoga was now taught from guru to student and used to gain insight.

During this time, there were three essential yoga paths:

BHAKTI YOGA – *the path of devotion. It refers to devotion to God or the highest consciousness in any manifestations. A loving relationship with God is developed through acts such as singing and reciting the name of God; this is seen as the easiest path to moksha.*

JNANA YOGA – *the path of knowledge. In Jnana yoga, theorizing gains insight into and understanding the spiritual aspect. Moksha is achieved by understanding that Brahman and Atman are the same.*

KARMA YOGA – *the path of selfless action. The practice of selfless acts unites practitioners with the highest consciousness. You work and help others without taking credit for it. Being fully present in your work makes you a tool for the universe.*

The Bhagavad Gita, seen as a summary of the Upanishads, takes place on the battlefield. Krishna tells Arjuna that he will win the war by following the three yoga paths – Bhakti, Karma, and Jnana yoga.

CLASSICAL YOGA

The critical work for classical yoga (200CE-400CE) was Patanjali's Yoga Sutras – a verse book and one of the six philosophical paths within Hinduism today. Yoga now had its philosophy. Patanjali divided yoga into eight steps with a focus on concentration. In this context, asanas meant a stable and comfortable position. The physical body was to be steady and immobile during meditation to avoid distraction.

According to Patanjali, an individual comprises Prakriti (matter) and Purusha (soul). Here, the goal of yoga is to stop identifying with the human body, and in doing so, the soul will be liberated and allowed to reunite with the Brahman (universe).

POST-CLASSICAL YOGA

All forms of yoga that came into being after Patanjali are categorized as post-classical yoga (500CE-700CE). Here, tantrism has a significant influence. Unlike in classical yoga, the body and the mind were now seen as one. Previously, the body had been experienced as an obstacle, and meditation was used as a means to the body and worldly matters. This era focused on returning to the origin of yoga: to rejuvenate the body and learn to master it to awaken Kundalini's power. According to tantrism, Kundalini's energy exists in every human being but as a dormant potential; this became the basis of Hatha yoga and the renaissance of tantra. Hatha Yoga Pradipika is an essential work in post-classical yoga.

MODERN/CONTEMPORARY YOGA

Swami Vivekananda (1863-1902) was a Hindu theorist and spiritual leader. He was a student of Sri Ramakrishna and founded the Ramakrishna Mission in 1897. There, they carried out extensive work in healthcare, provided disaster relief, and trained people, among other things. In 1898, Vivekananda attended the World's Fair in the United States, where he introduced Hinduism, which came to play an essential role in the invasion of yoga in the West.

Indra Devi (1899-2001), a German yogi, is another person who played an essential role in the development of yoga. Indra is seen as the First Lady of yoga. At the time, yoga was primarily studied and practiced by men. Indra was active in the yoga industry for sixty years; she taught many different nationalities and has dramatically inspired yogis worldwide. Indra was the first to open a yoga studio in the USA in 1947.

Today's most famous tantric yogi is probably the Dalai Lama.

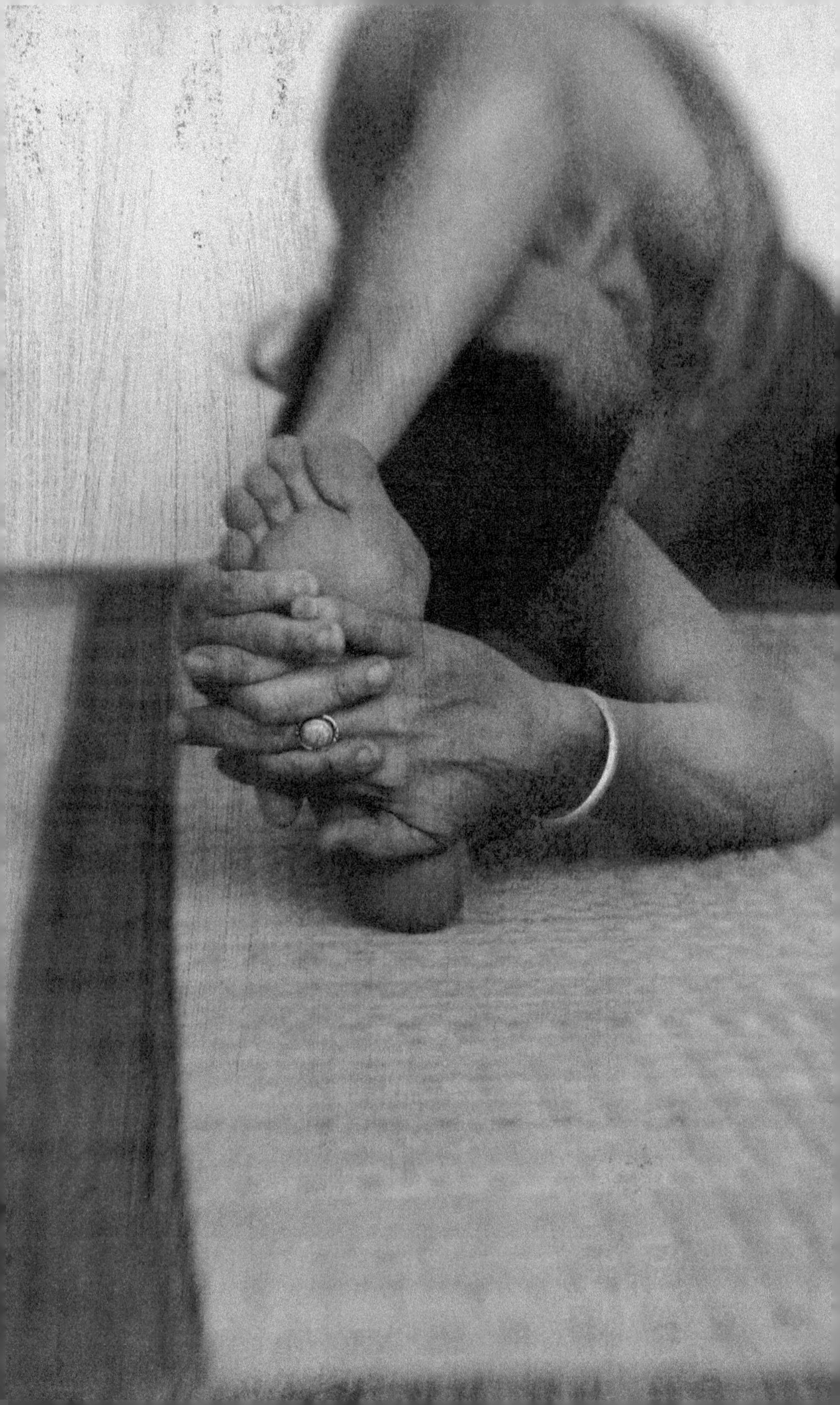

EVOLUTION OF YOGA THROUGH THE 36 TANTRA TATTWAS

36 TANTRA TATTWAS

Man is an image of the universe. The universe is the macrocosm, and man is the microcosm. Everything that is created and that we can see can also be invisible. It comes down to density and goes from the unmanifested to the manifested.

The thirty-six tantra tattwas describe creation from pure consciousness (Shiva) to matter (Shakti); this is represented by thirty-six steps, thirty-six manifestations, of energy that goes from the fine to the rough.

Everything has its beginning in the macrocosm, where there is pure consciousness. There was a densification of consciousness/energy. A vibration was heard – spandam, the sound of Aum, and thus Shakti was manifested.

5 SHIVA TATTWAS

Macrocosm structure

SHIVA
The timeless, eternal space

SHAKTI
The manifested time

ICHA
Will

JNANA
Knowledge

KRIYA
Movement

6 VIDYA TATTWAS

MAYA
Illusion

KALAA
Contraction of KRIYA

VIDYA
Contraction of JNANA

RAGA
Contraction of ICCHA

KALAA
Contraction of Shakti

NIYATI – *contraction* **CHICCHAKTI** *(Shiva)*

25 ATMA TATTWAS
Microcosm; man

PURUSHA	PRAKRITI
Shiva	*Shakti*

BUDDHI *– intellect, insight;*
SATTVIC GUNA contr. of JNANA

AHAMKARA *– ego;*
RAJASIC GUNA contraction of ICCHA

MANAS *– thoughts;*
TAMASIC GUNA contraction of KRIYA

5 JNANENDRIYAS
Sound, touch, sight, taste, smell (sense organs, sattvic)

5 KARMENDRIYAS
Speech, feeling, walking, emptying (toilet), sneezing (locomotor system, rajasic)

5 TANMANTRA
Sound, taste, shape, smell, touch (sensory attributes, tamasic)

5 MAHA BHUTAS

PRITHVI	APAS	AGNI	VAYU	AKASHA
Soil	*Water*	*Fire*	*Air*	*Space*

HATHA YOGA

THE YOGA OF BODY CONTROL

Much literature and texts refer to Hatha yoga, most written between 500CE and 1400CE. Hatha Yoga Pradipika by Yogi Swatmarama is one of the most famous. References to Hatha yoga are even made in the Upanishads and Puranas, written long before Buddhism (about 500 BCE). Traces of Hatha yoga have also been found in pre-Columbian culture in America. Even today, giant stone figures in St. Augustine in South America represent Hatha yoga asanas.

Hatha yoga is associated with Gorakhnath, a leading guru in Hatha yoga (approx. 500 CE-1100 CE). Gorakhnath was a disciple of Matsyendranatha, the first guru in Hatha yoga. Matsya means fish.

Buddha and Mahavir, the founders of the Jain sect, were two important figures in India around 500 BCE. At that time, man's spiritual development had been ongoing for centuries.

Two of the Buddha's teachings became known worldwide: Vipassana and Anapanasati. For these, the Buddha created a system called the Eightfold Path. This system deals with ethics and correct livelihood and has remarkable similarities to Raja Yoga's yamas and niyamas. Meditation became a popular method of spiritual development. However, they had no preparatory steps for meditation and eventually began to try the Buddha's system. Meditation was considered the highest path, but it was acknowledged that some preparations were required before practitioners could meditate.

Five hundred years after the time of the Buddha, a Buddhist university was established in Nalanda, Bihar, India. It was called the Hinayana system and was an orthodox Buddhist system.

At the same time, another university was established in Vikram Shila, Bihar, India. It became a learning center espousing the Mahayana tradition. They disagreed with the orthodox interpretation of the Buddha's teachings, viewing the Hinayana system as a deviation from the Buddha's teachings. The Mahayana tradition was founded by a group of liberal Buddhists who now began to embrace tantric thinking and philosophy.

After the fall of Buddhism in India (300 CE-500 CE), some great yogis wanted to return to the original doctrine of yoga and tantrism. Matsyendranatha and Goraknatha were two of these. They thought the essence of the principle had been forgotten and misunderstood by many. They separated Hatha and Raja yoga from the tantric rituals and developed the most useful, practical exercises in yoga and the tantric system. It also became necessary to reintroduce a proper meditation system. In this way, Hatha yoga was established. Matsyendranatha founded the Natha order.

To cleanse the body and its elements before meditation is the foundation of Hatha yoga.

In Hatha yoga, body and mind are seen as one and equally important.

THE FIVE ELEMENTS OF HATHA YOGA:

ASANAS

In Raja yoga, asanas refer to a comfortable and steady position. Hatha yoga asanas are specific postures that help open our energy channels and centers. Hatha yogis discovered they also gained control over the mind through reasonable body control. Therefore, asanas are put at the forefront of Hatha yoga.

PRANAYAMAS

Breathing influences the flow of prana in our nadis (energy channels). Breathwork is a method through which breathing exercises activate, regulate, and purify our life energy in the energy body. You get a higher degree of power and increase your consciousness.

MUDRAS

Mudra can be translated as posture or gesture. Various energy points are stimulated through mudras, affecting our body and mind. Mudras can influence your mood and deepen your concentration and consciousness. You hold on to and redirect prana through mudras, which would otherwise disappear from the body. In this way, mudras also play an important role in awakening Kundalini Shakti.

BANDHAS

Traditionally, bandhas are classified as part of mudras. Bandhas are often combined with mudras and pranayamas, but they are an essential group of exercises in their own right. Bandha means lock, which describes movement and its effect on our energy body. Prana is locked in specific areas of the body, and the flow of prana to the sushumna nadi is controlled, which develops our spiritual awakening.

SHATKARMAS

Shatkarmas are a series of purification processes divided into six groups. These aim to create harmony between ida and pingala nadi to achieve mental and physical balance and purity. Purification processes are also used before breathing exercises to expel toxins from the body.

HATHA YOGA PRADIPIKA

Hatha Yoga Pradipika is a classic textbook on Hatha yoga. It was written in the fifteenth century by Swami Svatmarama, a Swami Gorakhnath disciple. Hatha Yoga Pradipika is thus the oldest preserved Hatha yoga text and one of the three classical texts, next to Gheranda Samhita and Shiva Samhita.

The book contains a total of three hundred and ninety verses. Of these, about forty are dedicated to asanas, about one hundred to pranayamas, one-hundred-and-fifty to mudras, bandhas, and shatkarmas, and the rest to pratyahara, dharana, dhyana and samadhi. The book consists of four chapters:

1.) Asana: Svatmarama honors his teachers and explains why he wrote the book and who he wrote it for. He describes how and where yoga should be practiced. Svatmarama then describes fifteen asanas and gives recommendations for eating habits.

2.) Pranayama: Svatmarama addresses the connections between breathing, mind, Kundalini, bandha, nadi, and prana. He then describes six karmas and eight kumbhakas.

3.) Mudras: The author describes ten different mudras.

4.) Samadhi: Svatmarama discusses samadhi, laya, nada, two mudras, and the four steps of yoga.

Hatha Yoga Pradipika is dedicated to Lord Adinatha, another name for Shiva (a Hindu god of destruction and renewal), and is believed to have revealed the mysteries of Hatha yoga to his divine consort Parvati.

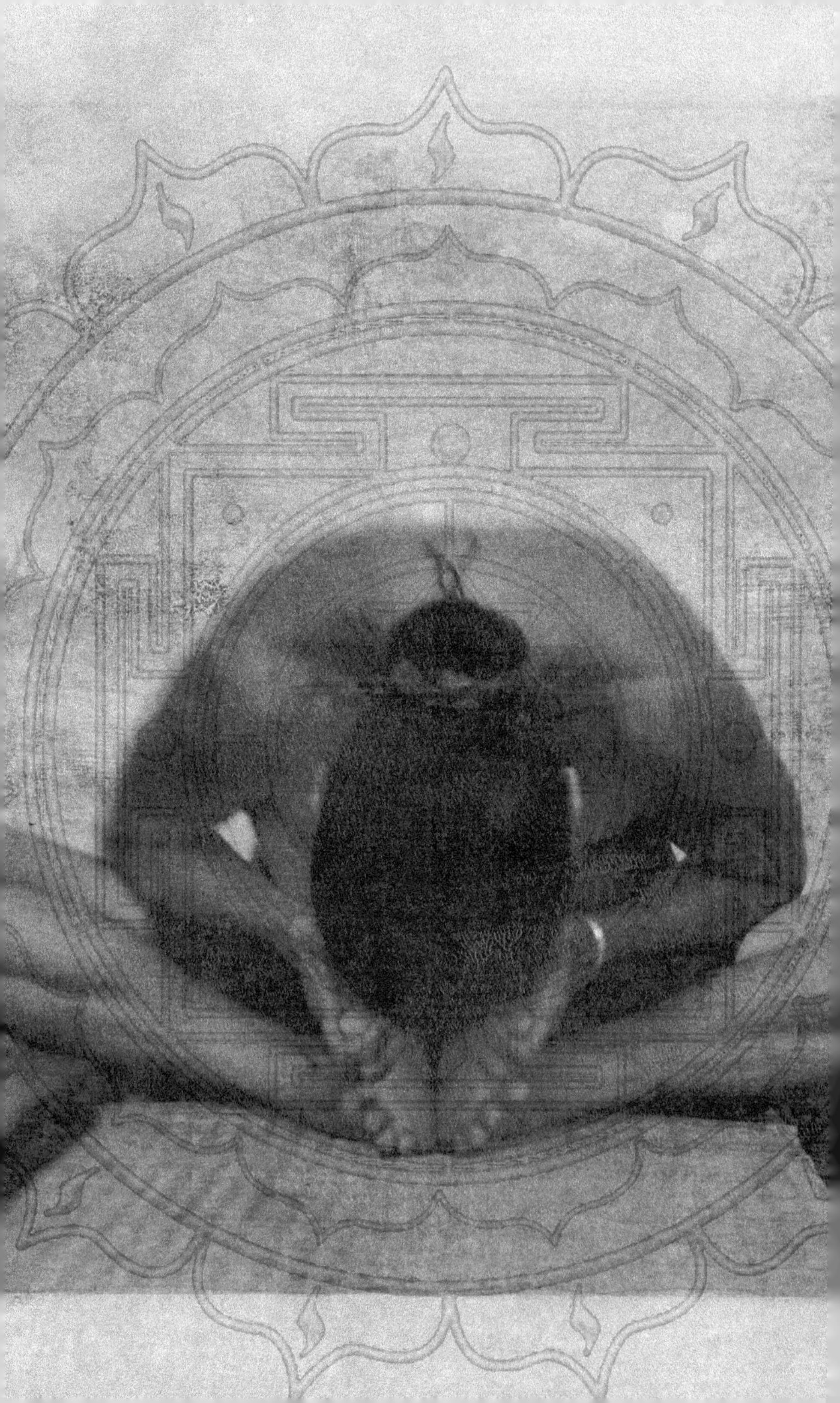

ADVANCED HATHA YOGA

OUR FIVE SHEATHS

Our physical body, the three bodies of the astral body, and our innermost interior.

Hatha yoga teaches that we consist of five sheaths or bodies:

ANNAMAYA KOSHA

Physical body.

PRANAMAYA KOSHA

Energy body.

MANAMAYA KOSHA

Mental body.

VIGYANAMAYA KOSHA

Wisdom Body.

ANANDAMAYA KOSHA

Bliss body (pure consciousness of true self).

The energy body, the mental body, and the wisdom body form the astral body.

NADIS – IDA AND PINGALA AND SUSHUMNA NADI

Pranamaya kosha – our energy body – consists of about seventy-two thousand nadis (subtle channels through which prana flows). It is the energy body that gives us life. The three most important nadis are ida, pingala, and sushumna nadi, of which sushumna nadi is the most important.

Ida nadi flows from the left side of the spine and controls mental energy. It is associated with the parasympathetic nervous system. Pingala nadi flows along the right side of the divide and controls our physical body. It is associated with the sympathetic nervous system. Sushumna nadi, the most important of the three, flows along the entire spine and channels the spiritual energy.

Ida and pingala nadi flow from the root chakra and cross the sushumna nadi at four places in the body to finally unite at the eyebrow center. Ida nadi then goes out through the left nostril and pingala nadi through the right.

We can regulate the body's energies through asanas, and when ida and pingala nadi flow simultaneously, sushumna nadi opens. Kundalini Shakti can begin to travel upwards and activate our chakra system, illuminating our brain's dormant parts. Usually, we use about twenty percent of our brain capacity. Special siddhis, paranormal abilities, arise on our path to activating a more significant part of the brain. You become a Siddha. However, these abilities are not the ultimate goal.

HA + THA

Ha – pingala nadi – the sun stands for the sympathetic nervous system, and tha – ida nadi – the moon stands for the parasympathetic nervous system.

OUR SUBTLE ENERGY BODY WITH FIVE PRANA VAYUS

Our five bodies interact with each other and create a whole. The breathing exercises mainly affect our energy body – pranamaya kosha, which comprises five different types of sub-pranas. These five prana vayus (wind) are prana, apana, samana, udana and vyana. The link also binds the bodies together and affects us in all directions. If we calm the body with breathing, we also calm the mind and vice versa, which you probably have experienced during your yoga practice.

PRANA

In this context, prana does not refer to the cosmic prana but to the flow of energy that controls the thorax area between the larynx and the diaphragm. This area is linked to the heart and respiratory system, along with the muscles and nerves that activate them. It is this power that makes us draw inward breath.

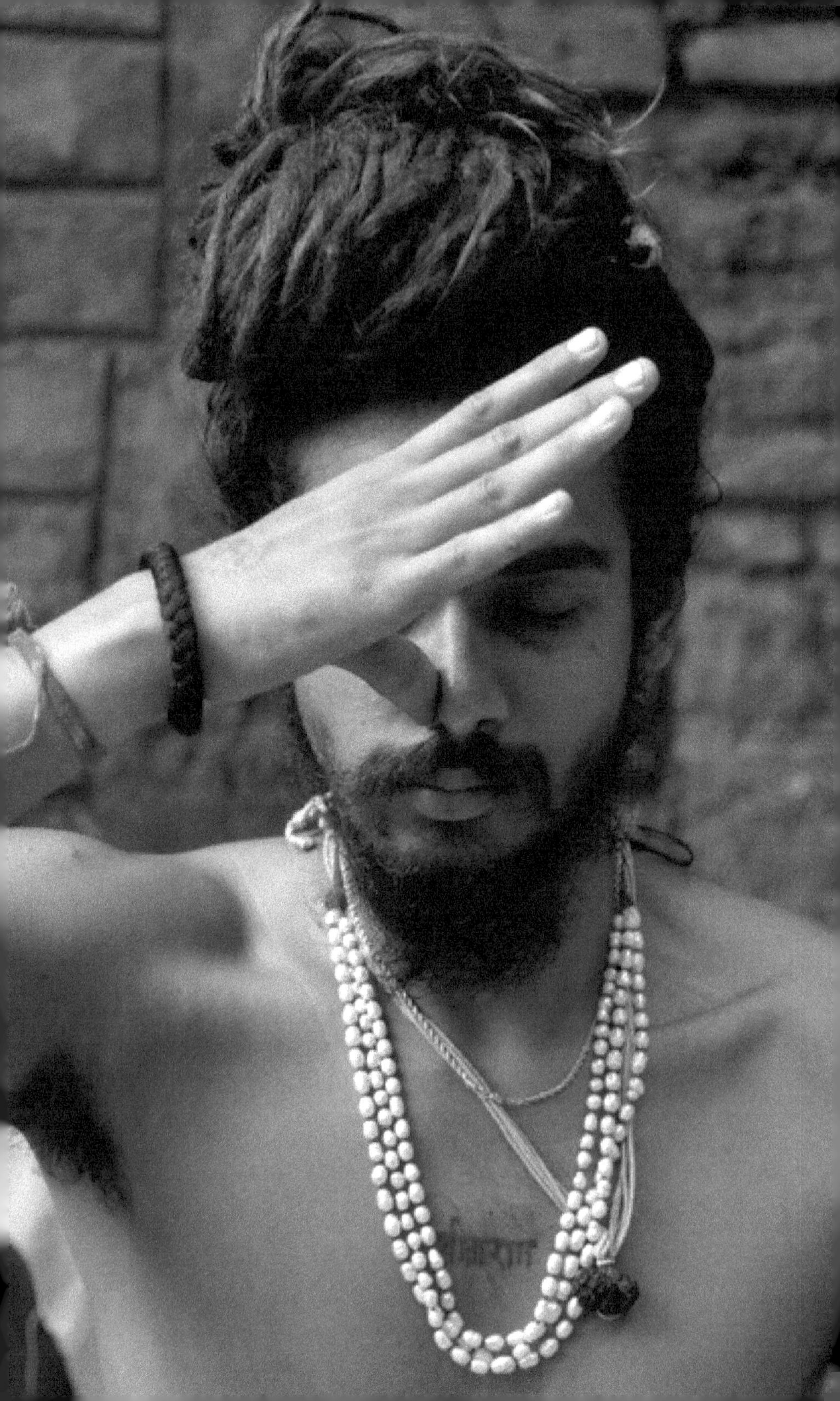

APANA

Apana controls the abdomen and the area under the navel, providing energy to the intestines, kidneys, rectum, and genitals. It affects the expulsion of waste products in the body and is the force that makes us exhale.

SAMANA

Samana is located between the heart and the navel. It activates and controls the digestive system. Samana is responsible for the transformation; physically, the transformation refers to the very distribution of nutrients in the body, and evolutionarily, it relates to Kundalini power and the development of our consciousness.

UDANA

Udana controls the area of the neck and head. It activates all our sensory receptors, including eyes, tongue, nose, and ears. Udana activates and balances muscles, ligaments, nerves, and joints in our arms and legs. It is responsible for our posture, sensory attention, and ability to interact with the outside world.

VYANA

Vyana permeates the whole body. It regulates and controls all our movements and coordinates all sub-pranas in the body.

In addition to the most critical sub-pranas, five smaller pranas are called upa-pranas. These five are naga, koorma, krikara, devadatta, and dhananjaya. Naga is responsible for belching and hiccups; koorma opens our eyes and makes us blink; krikara creates hunger, thirst, sneezing, and coughing; devadatta generates sleep and yawn; and dhananjaya activates when we die, and our body begins to break down.

PRANA AND LIFESTYLE

Our lifestyle has a significant impact on our energy body and its prana. Physical activity such as exercise, work, sleep, food, and sexual relationships affect the distribution and flow of prana in our body. Emotions, thoughts, and fantasies affect our bodies even more. An unbalanced lifestyle, poor diet, and stress break down and block the flow of prana. It results in feeling drained of energy. When energy becomes low in one of our sub-pranas, the very area of the body that the prana controls is affected and may result in illness. Breathing exercises can prevent this by balancing or increasing the energy in our energy body.

ASANA

There is a definition of asanas – Stirham Sukham Asana – in Patanjali's Yoga Sutras, which means steady or comfortable position. They wanted to develop their ability to sit still for a long time because it was a prerequisite for meditation.

In Hatha yoga, however, it was discovered that specific postures, asanas, opened up energy channels and mental centers in the body. You have better body control and could thus also develop control over the mind, thoughts, and energies. Yoga asanas became a tool for achieving higher consciousness and provided a stable foundation to explore the body, mind, and breathing.

Initially, there were eight-million-four-hundred-thousand different asanas. These represent as many lives an unenlightened person must be reborn into before becoming enlightened. Rishis and yogis scaled down the number to the few hundred known today. Of these, the eighty-four most important asanas were then highlighted. Thirty-five asanas have a direct impact on our chakras. The others purify and regulate our nadis. Asanas create a balance between body and mind and a flow in the sushumna.

Rishis studied the animals and noticed how they lived harmoniously with their bodies and surroundings. By mimicking the animals' movements and postures, hormone secretion in the body was affected. During deep meditation, they observed how different poses affected the body and the mind.

Prana, the vital energy (life energy), permeates our entire body—a poor flow of prana in the body results in stiffness and an accumulation of toxins. When prana flows freely, these toxins are removed, and the body becomes soft and supple. Even the most challenging postures are easy to perform because when the amount of prana increases in the body, pranic intuition is achieved. An intuitive sense of how to perform asanas, mudras, and pranayamas follows.

Hatha yoga increases overall health and activates our energy centers by balancing the nervous system.

Asanas in Hatha yoga release tensions that arise as knots in our muscles. By removing these tensions from the body, we also release tensions from the mind. It makes us feel better in general and releases underlying and hidden energy that lies latent.

Thus, asanas are more than exercise. They are techniques that place the body in different positions to promote awareness, relaxation, concentration, and meditation. Part of this process is to develop a good physique through stretching, stimulation of prana, and massage of the glands and internal organs.

Asanas are divided into three groups: beginners, intermediate and advanced. It is optional to complete all the exercises in each group. Daily practice of a tailor-made program will have the most significant effect.

Those who have never practiced yoga should perform asanas for beginners. These have a more significant effect on beginners' bodies than advanced exercises. These exercises prepare the body and mind for more advanced exercises and meditation and help improve physical health.

The intermediate asanas are for those who can efficiently complete the exercises for beginners. These require greater concentration, steadiness, and coordination with movement and breathing.

Advanced asanas are for those with well-developed body control, muscles, and nervous system. You should be able to master the intermediate exercises without problem. It is essential to take your time and start these exercises early enough.

DYNAMIC AND STATIC ASANAS

Dynamic asanas increase flexibility and circulation in the body. They soften muscles, release knots and energy blockages, and remove stagnant blood. These asanas are most important for the beginner. To start work with the chakra system, for example, blockages must first be released; otherwise, the energy may flow the wrong way in the energy body. Dynamic asanas and vinyasa process our physical body; they take us deeper and prepare us for the more static asanas. Hatha yoga often starts with a lot of movement and gradual-

ly lets the vibrations subside into stillness and silence. It has much to do with moving from the rough to the fine – from the body to the mind – and knowing how yoga affects our doshas through Ayurveda.

VINYASA

Dynamic asanas are often synchronized with breathing. When we do that, it's called vinyasa—a flow where movements and breathing interact.

Vinyasa aims to increase the internal cleansing and detoxification of the body. Breathing synchronized with movement warms the blood. Thick blood is often unhealthy and causes diseases. The heat from vinyasa cleanses the blood and makes it thinner so it can circulate better in the body and around our joints, reducing pain.

Where there is poor circulation in the body, pain usually occurs. The heated blood also passes through all the internal organs. It transports impurities and diseases removed from the body with our increased amount of sweat during the yoga session.

Sweat is an essential by-product of vinyasa. It is only through our sweat that diseases can leave the body and be purified, in the same way, that gold is melted to eliminate its impurities. Yoga boils the blood and transports contaminants and toxins to the surface, which are then removed with the help of sweat. If you practice vinyasa often, the body becomes healthy, strong, clean, and shiny like gold.

With the body cleansed, it is possible to cleanse the nervous system and sense organs.

STATIC ASANAS

Static and, above all, inverted asanas have the most profound effect on our energy body and our chakra system. These require greater flexibility and are suited for more experienced practitioners. Remaining in the position for a few minutes has a more powerful effect on the glands, prana, chakras, and internal organs. The mind becomes calm and prepares the individual for meditation. Some static asanas are beneficial for reaching pratyahara.

TRISTHANA

Tristhana means three areas to pay attention to: postures (position, stretching, and relaxation), breath, and gazing point. They are always performed in conjunction with each other.

Asanas cleanse, strengthen, and soften the body. We cleanse the nervous system when we breathe with rechaka and puraka, a steady and even inhalation and exhalation at the same pace. Drishti is the place you look at during yoga practice.

There are nine different ones: the tip of the nose, eyebrow center, navel, thumbs, hands, feet, right and left side, up to the sky. Drishi purifies, captures, and stabilizes the mind.

ADVICE FOR THE PRACTICE OF ASANAS:

BREATH

According to Hatha yoga, two components are needed to cleanse the body internally: the elements air and fire. Fire, our life force, is located at the solar plexus in the body and is generated by the Manipura chakra. Air is required for fire to burn, hence the importance of proper breathing in yoga. Long, even breaths increase the internal fire in the body, which heats the blood for physical purification and burns up impurities in the nervous system. As the inner fire increases in strength, so does our digestive system, health, and longevity. Uneven breathing creates an imbalance in our physical body and its signaling system, weakening our immune system. We risk becoming ill in the long run – according to Hatha yoga, we tolerate stress and toxins less.

Another critical component to increase the inner fire is moola and uddiyana bandha: root and stomach locks. They increase the effect of breathing, keep it inside the body longer, encapsulate the energy, and provide light, strength, and health to the body. According to Hatha yoga, six toxins in the body surround our spiritual heart. The light in our heart is obscured by these six poisons: kama, krodha, moha, lobha, matsarya, and mada. They are desire, anger, delusion, greed, envy and sloth. When we practice Hatha yoga for an extended period with power, determination, and proper breathing, the increasing heat in the body will burn up these six toxins, and the light in our interior will shine through.

Breathing through the nose (unless otherwise stated) and coordinating breathing with movement is essential. But never force yourself to breathe through your nose. If you need to breathe through your mouth, do it. Your fine energy channels can be damaged otherwise, and the energy will flow the wrong way in the energy body. If you are panting, wait until you can breathe through your nose again more quickly.

CONSCIOUSNESS

The purpose of asanas is to influence and create harmony in all aspects of man: physical, mental, emotional, pranic, and spiritual. By performing asanas consciously, all these parts are affected. One should be aware of body sensations, movement, and posture on its own and in coordination with breathing, the flow of prana, focus on the chakra and witness thoughts and feelings that come up.

RELAXATION

You can lie down in shavasana at any time for rest or contemplation. Notice how it feels in the body.

SERIES

You always begin with shatkarmas (purification processes), such as nasal rinsing (jala neti). Then you perform asanas, pranayamas, pratyahara, and dharana (concentration/quiet the mind), leading to dhyana (meditation). You can also add both breathing exercises and meditation before asanas. It fulfills a function – especially at the beginning of your yoga practice that you go from the outside in (see the text about our five bodies) before you intuitively know what, when, and how to do it.

OPPOSITION

It is essential to have a structure in the program to balance the body and nervous system. A backward bending and vice versa should always follow a forward bending position. However, this does not apply to yoga rehabilitation.

TIME

Asanas can be practiced at any time of the day, provided you have not eaten a few hours prior. That said, practicing just before sunrise and sunset is recommended. The time of day just before daylight is called Brahma muhurta (the divine time – God's time). The atmosphere is still clean, the stomach and intestines inactive, and the mind still. The most favorable time is before sunrise and sunset, but do not be too ambitious. A yoga session during the day is better than having no session.

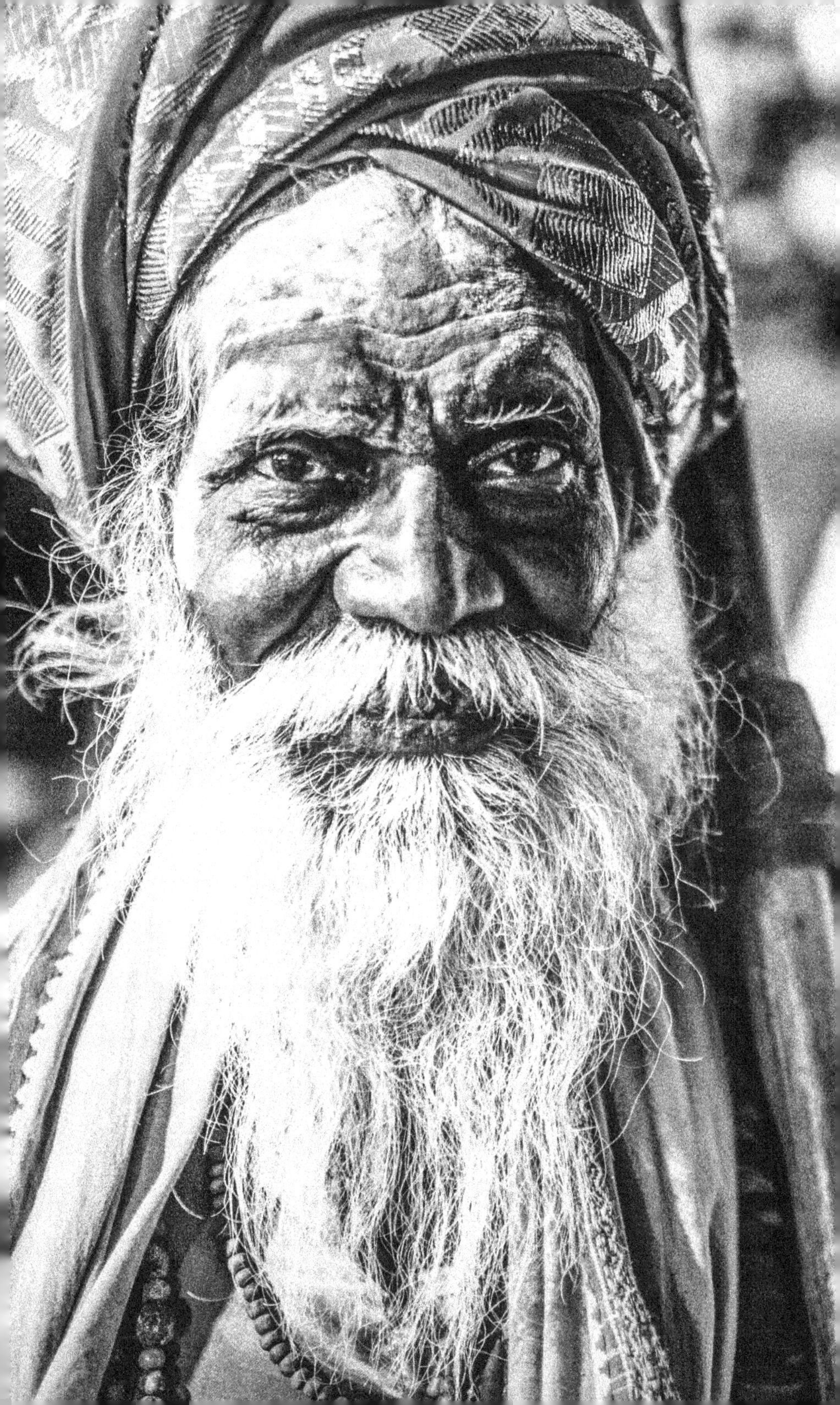

PLACE

One should find a secluded place that is tidy, clean, quiet, and peaceful. No furniture or objects should be in the way. You can also practice outdoors in a comfortable and beautiful place, not in the cold and wind, where the air is unclean, or in the scorching sun.

CHOICE OF YOGA MAT

Use a mat made of natural materials. It has the most beneficial effect on our pranic currents. Choose a yoga mat you can use for many years to come of the best quality; the prana is stored in the mat and has a beneficial effect on the body. So, take care of your yoga mat and treat it tenderly. Make sure that you can lie on it comfortably and that it is not too small or too thin so that the surface is felt if you, e.g., standing on the head. It should be damping but, at the same time, provide a good grip. A good yoga mat will last at least ten years or longer, so don't be stingy with yourself. Treat yourself to a premium yoga mat of the right size and with the right feeling.

CLOTHES

Wear loose and comfortable clothes, remove jewelry, and be barefoot so you do not slip.

SHOWER

Try to take a cold shower before the session to wake the body up. After the session, wait to shower so you do not unnecessarily cool down your body too quickly and lose the healing effect of yoga.

LOO
Empty the stomach.

DIET
There are no strict rules regulating what food to eat. However, a natural diet in moderate amounts is recommended so that not all energy is used to digest food. A vegetarian diet is not essential, but it is recommended. The stomach should be filled half with food, a quarter with water, and a quarter should be left empty. However, do not drink water during the practice as it draws blood and energy to the stomach and cools down your energy body. Also, wait two to three hours to practice yoga after eating so it does not feel uncomfortable during the session.

PERFORMANCE
Asanas are performed softly and gently in three steps:

Awareness of the body, movement, and thoughts creates calm, balance, and focus, leading to a state of harmony in the body.

Awareness of breathing. Synchronize movement with brea-

thing. The action becomes calmer, and brain waves become slower. You become relaxed and gain an increased understanding.

Awareness of the flow of prana can be experienced as tingles in the body. The feeling is developed through regular practice. You become mentally calm, focused, and emotionally receptive.

Asanas are also divided into three parts:

Starting poses.
Implementation.
Final poses.

IMPORTANT
A physician should be consulted before performing asanas in the event of any injury or illness.

Asanas must never hurt joints, complex parts, or ligaments during practice.

Inverted asanas should be avoided during gas formation (toxins can reach the brain), late pregnancy, and menstruation (the cycle can be disrupted). Never sunbathe immediately following yoga practice to avoid overheating.

PRANAYAMAS

Pranayama means breathing technique or breathing control and originates from the words prana – (life force or life energy), yama (discipline or power), and ayama (extension, restraint, or expansion). Pranayamas are divided into puraka (inhalation), kumbhaka (retention of breath), and rechaka (exhalation). Kumbhaka, in turn, is divided into bahir (the retention of breath immediately following exhalation) and antar (holding your breath inside after inhaling). In yogic writings, kevala kumbhaka is also mentioned. It is an advanced yogic condition where breathing via the lungs stops spontaneously, and energy (prana) seeps through the pores in the body's cells.

HEALTH AND BREATHING

Breathing is the most important function we have in the body. It affects the activity of every single cell, including the brain and its operations. A person breathes about fifteen breaths per minute and about twenty-thousand-six hundred breaths daily. Most live incompletely, using only a tiny part of our lungs' capacity. The breathing then becomes shallow, and the body becomes poor in oxygen and prana, which are necessary to maintain good health.

Rhythmic, deep, and slow breathing encourages and is encouraged by a calm and satisfied state of mind. Irregular and uneven breathing disrupts the brain's rhythm, leading to physical, emotional, and mental blockages. It, in turn, causes internal conflicts, an unbalanced personality, a disordered lifestyle, and illness. You build a regular breathing pattern and break this vicious circle through breathing exercises. We learn to regain control of breathing and rebuild our body and mind's natural, relaxed rhythm.

Despite being an unconscious process, you can turn breathing into a conscious process at any time; it creates a link between the unconscious and conscious parts of our mind. The energy that is absorbed by neurotic and unconscious mental patterns can be released with the help of breathing exercises. The energy can then be used on something creative and joyful.

BREATHING AND LIFE

Ancient yogis and rishis studied nature in detail. They noted that animals with slow breathing had a long lifespan, and animals with fast breathing only lived for a few years. Through this observation, they realized how crucial slow breathing is for longevity. Physically, breathing is directly linked to the heart. Slow breathing keeps the heart strong, which leads to a longer life. Deep breathing also increases the absorption of energy in our energy body, which increases mobility, vitality, and well-being.

BREATHING EXERCISES AND THE SPIRITUAL SEARCH

Breathing exercises build a healthy body by releasing blockages in the energy body, increasing the absorption and retention of prana. A calm and quiet mind is a prerequisite for spiritual exercises. In many breathing exercises, kumbhaka (retention of breath) controls the flow of prana, calms the mind, and controls the thought process. When the mind is calmed down, and prana can flow freely through our nadis and chakras, the development of our consciousness is enabled; it, in turn, can lead us to higher dimensions of spiritual experiences.

COMMON ADVICE

Contraindications. Breathing exercises should not be practiced during illness. However, lighter exercises such as conscious or abdominal breathing in shavasana are still acceptable.

TIME

The best time for breathing exercises is in the morning before sunrise. The body is calm, and the mind is still, as it has not yet had time to absorb many impressions from its surroundings. If this is impossible, the second-best time is in the evening when the sun goes down. Soothing breathing exercises are good to do before falling asleep. Try breathing exercises simultaneously and in the same place every day. Regular practice builds strength and willpower.

HYGIENE

Take a bath or shower before practicing pranayamas. At least wash your hands, face, and feet. Please wait at least half an hour to bathe after completing breathing exercises; it is to allow the body temperature to normalize.

FOOD

Eat your breakfast after completing the practice, or wait three to four hours after eating to practice. With food in the stomach, pressure forms on the diaphragm and lungs, making breathing difficult to deeply and completely. It hinders the use of the total capacity of the lungs.

When you start practicing breathing exercises, you may experience constipation and a decrease in urine. If this occurs, reduce salt and spices, and drink plenty of water. Should you encounter an anxious stomach and an increase in urine, take a break from practice for a few days.

PLACE

Practice in a place where you can find peace and where it is clean. The area should be well-ventilated, but not so you are sitting in a draft. Avoid direct sunlight as it may cause overheating.

BREATH

Always breathe through your nose unless otherwise instructed. The air must be able to flow freely through both nostrils.

SEQUENCE

*Breathing exercises are done after shatkarmas, often after as-
anas, and before meditation, but can also be practiced before
asanas. Nadi shodana should be included in each breathing
exercise. Lie down in shavasana for a few minutes after completing the asanas.*

SITTING POSITION

*A comfortable sitting position is necessary to keep the body
and breathing stable during the exercises. The body should
be as relaxed as possible with a straight spine and neck. The
mat should be made of natural material. If you cannot sit
comfortably in a meditation position for a long time, you can
sit against a wall with outstretched legs or on a chair with a
straight backrest.*

*Avoid exertion. It is important to remember not to exert too
much effort when doing breathing exercises. Take your time
to advance. Only move on to the next step once you feel enti-
rely comfortable with a routine. Keeping your breath inside/
out is only achieved as long as it feels comfortable.*

SIDE EFFECTS

*Various physical and mental symptoms can occur in nor-
mally healthy people. Physical symptoms occur as a result
of the detoxification of toxins. Feelings like tingling, heat
and cold, lightness, and heaviness may occur. These are*

usually temporary. Energy levels may increase or fluctuate, and interests may change. If these changes create problems, you should seek the guidance of a competent guru. Excessive pranayamas late at night can lead to sleeping problems and an extreme excess of energy the next day – what many wrongly describe as a Kundalini awakening or hypersensitivity. Pranayamas are powerful tools and should be treated with respect. Slightly simplified, you can say that through breathing exercises, agni (fire) is increased in us, and Manipura chakra at the navel increases its activity; it causes vayu (air) attached to the chakra above, Anahata, to be netted and expanded. As the air expands, so does the space within us (Akasha), and a more profound spiritual experience is reached. However, increasing the amount of vayu can lead to anxiety and worry, so you must end each session by reducing the excess of vata you have built up. Excessive practice can, in the worst case, lead to psychosis and delusions.

MUDRA/GESTURE

Mudra can be translated as posture or gesture. Various energy points that affect both body and mind are stimulated through mudras. Your mood is influenced, and your consciousness and ability to concentrate are increased. With the help of mudras, you can hold and control prana that would otherwise disappear from the body. Hence, mudras also play an important role in awakening Kundalini's energy. Mudras can be done as a single exercise or in combination with

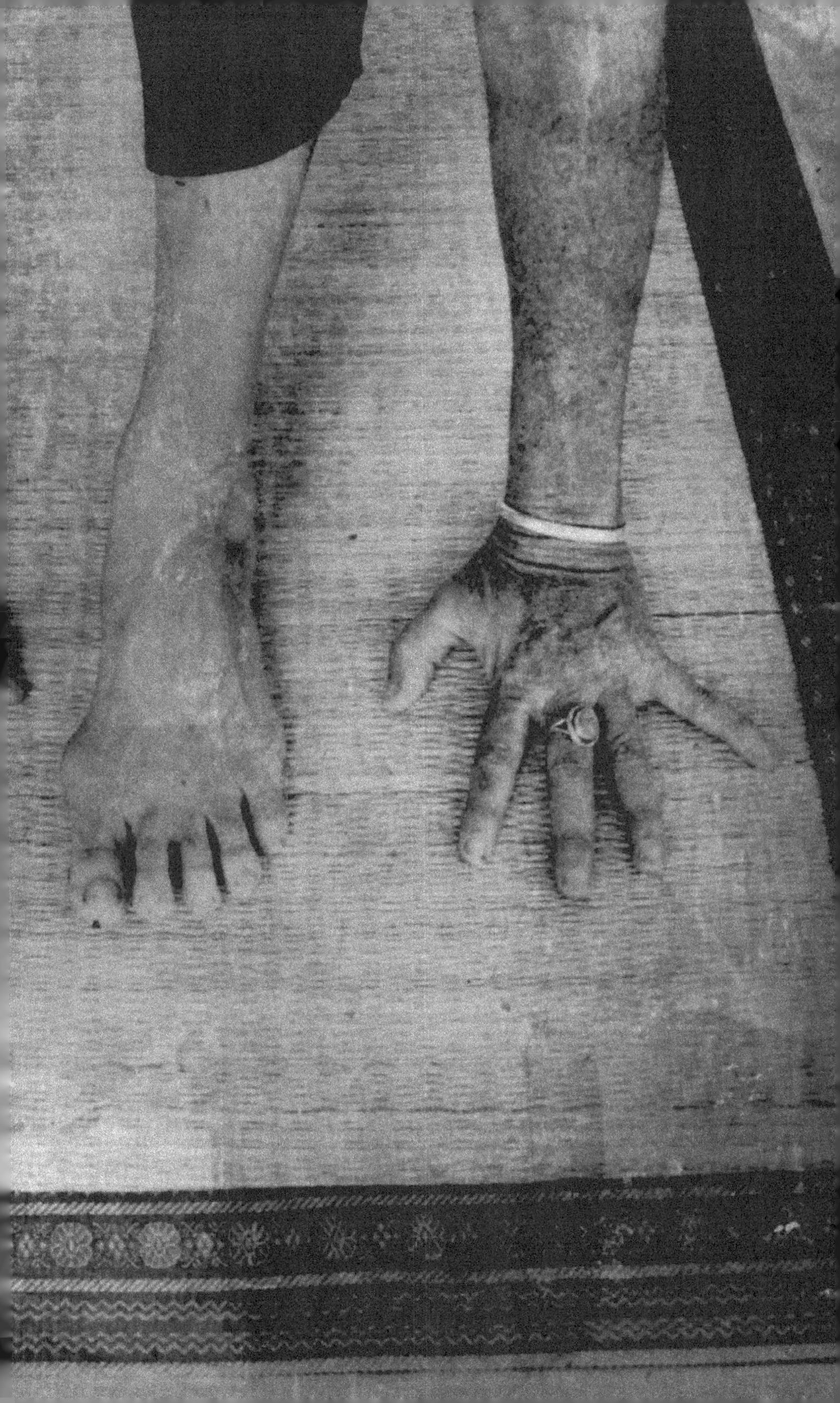

asanas, pranayamas, bandhas, and different visualization techniques.

In Hatha Yoga Pradipika, mudras are discussed as "yoganaga": a separate branch of yoga that requires a subtle presence. You often learn these techniques after you have become accustomed to and knowledgeable in asanas, pranayamas, and bandhas and when you have eliminated blockages from the body. Mudras are among the more advanced techniques that awaken our prana, chakras, and Kundalini Shakti, which can open up various siddhis (paranormal or mental forces) in the more advanced practitioners.

Mudras create a direct link between annamaya kosha (our physical body), manomaya kosha (our mental body), and pranamaya kosha (our energy body); it increases the feeling and awareness of the flow of prana in the body. A pranic balance is created in our koshas, and the subtle energy is directed to the higher chakras, promoting increased consciousness.

Our nadis and chakras radiate energy, which usually disappears from the body into our surroundings. By creating barriers within the body with the help of mudras, the energy is instead directed inwards. According to Tantric literature, when prana is kept in the body with the assistance of mudras, the mind becomes introverted, which leads to pratyahara

– withdrawal of our senses – as well as dharana (concentration).

Mudras can be divided into five different categories:

HASTA / HAND MUDRA

These lead the energy created in our hands back into the body. You create an energy path that flows from the brain to the hands and back again. If you know this process, an inner awareness is completed quickly. Mudras in this category are: jnana mudra, chin mudra, yoni mudra, bhairava mudra, and hridayamudra.

MANA / HEAD MUDRA

These techniques are essential to Kundalini yoga; many are meditation techniques. Here, you use eyes, ears, nose, tongue and lips. Mudras in this category are: shambhavi mudra, nasikagra drishti, khechari mudra, khaki mudra, bhujangini mudra, bhoochari mudra, akashi mudra, shanmukhi mudra, and unmani mudra.

KAYA MUDRA

These exercises are combined with asanas, breathing techniques, and concentration. Mudras in this category are: vipareeta karani mudra, pashinee mudra, prana mudra, yoga mudra, manduki mudra and tadagi mudra.

BANDHA / LOCK

These exercises combine mudras and bandhas. They charge the system with prana and prepare for the awakening of Kundalini Shakti. Techniques in this category are maha mudra, maha bheda mudra, and maha vedha mudra.

Adhara: these techniques direct the prana from the lower parts of the body to the brain. Techniques that use sexual energy belong to this group and are extremely powerful. Techniques in this category are ashwini mudra and vajroli/ sahajoli mudra.

MUDRAS AND OUR ELEMENTS

In the yogic tradition, our hands are like a map of our well-being. Different points in our hands are directly linked to other body parts and our psyche. We stimulate these points and energy paths by making various mudras or hand positions.

Like our surroundings, our physical body comprises five elements: earth, water, fire, air, and ether (space). Many people know the first four elements, but ether(space) is often unknown. Ether (space) is a subtle celestial energy high above our earth. In our body, ether is the space within us at the cellular level.

Imbalances in our elements weaken our immune system, leading to illness in the long run. These deficiencies or ine-qualities can be corrected by connecting different body parts in a specific way by mudras. Mudras create electromagnetic currents in the body, so-called energy loops. Each element is also associated with a chakra. When the element is balanced, the chakra is also affected and, in turn, affects the energy (vayu) that belongs to the chakra's area.

Finger	*Element/Tattwa*	*Chakra*	*Energy/Vayu*
Thumb	*Fire/agni*	*Manipura*	*Samana*
Index finger	*Air/vayu*	*Anahata*	*Prana*
Middle finger	*Ether/akasha*	*Vishuddhi*	*Udana*
The ring finger	*Earth/prithvi*	*Mooladhara*	*Apana*
Little finger	*Water/apas*	*Swadhisthana*	*Vyana*

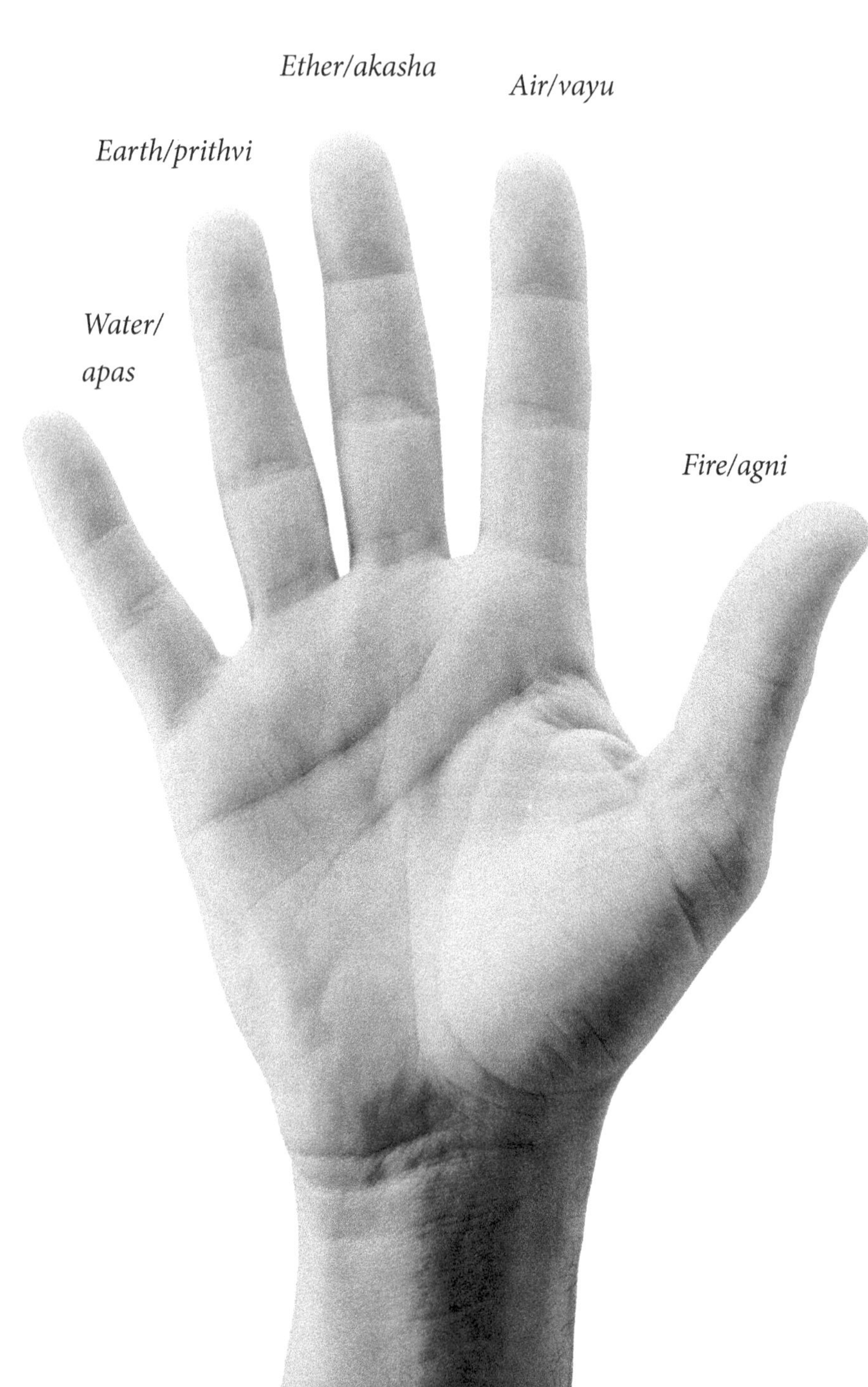

Ether/akasha
Air/vayu
Earth/prithvi
Water/
apas
Fire/agni

HASTA MUDRA PRANAYAMA

(4 four steps)

SEQUENCE

1. Chin mudra pranayama.

Sit in a comfortable meditation position. Extend the spine and neck. Place your hands, palms facing up, on your knees. Press your thumb against the index finger and let the other fingers point straight out. Sit still, close your eyes, and follow your natural breathing for a few minutes.

Chin mudra opens up the lower lobes of the lungs and stimulates apana vayu (prana that moves down from the navel to the perineum). Physically, it is responsible for the expulsion of toxins in the body.

Sit still and follow the breathing that moves in and out of the nose—two to three minutes.

2. Chin maya mudra pranayama.

Now fold in your fingers without touching your palms. Hold your thumb against your index finger.

Chin maya mudra pranayama opens up the middle lobes of our lungs and stimulates the samana vayu (prana that

*moves from left to right in the area around the abdomen).
Physically, it is responsible for digestion and our ability to as-
similate the nutrients in our food. On a subtle level, it affects
our ability to absorb (and learn from) life experiences.*

*Sit still and follow the breathing that moves in and out of the
nose—two to three minutes.*

3. Aadi mudra pranayama.

*Now grab the thumbs with your other fingers and place the
fists on the knees with the back of the hand up.*

*Aadi mudra pranayama opens the upper lobes of our lungs.
It stimulates the udana vayu (prana that moves upwards
towards the head and outwards in our extremities). Physically, it is responsible for healing and balancing our sense
organs. On a subtle level, it is responsible for balancing our
perception.*

*Sit still and follow the breathing that moves in and out of the
nose—two to three minutes.*

4. Brahma mudra pranayama.

*Hold the position of the hands, but turn them so that the
wrists are facing upwards and the knuckles are facing each*

other. Press your hands against your body level with your pelvis.

Brahma mudra pranayama opens up the whole lung. It opens up vyana vayu – the energy that makes us go on a bit longer, the last boost. It balances and starts our other pranas in the body when they become low. It revitalizes the whole system. Sit still and follow the breathing that moves in and out of the nose—two to three minutes.

BANDHA AND GRANTHI

Traditionally, bandhas are classified as part of mudras. In Hatha Yoga Pradipika and old tantric texts, mudras, and bandhas are seen as a whole; they are not separated. Bandhas are linked to mudras and to pranayamas. Bandhas are a technique that creates a unique lock in the body.

The word bandha means to hold or lock in Sanskrit. It describes the physical effect created in the body and the retention of prana. Bandhas lock the energy into specific body parts and control the flow to the sushumna nadi to create a spiritual awakening.

Bandhas should be learned as a separate technique before practicing them with mudras and pranayamas.

There are four locking techniques: jalandhara, moola, uddiyana, and maha bandha. Maha is a combination of the first three. These three bandhas directly impact our three mental points (granthis) in the body. Moola bandha is associated with Brahma granthi, uddiyana bandha with Vishnu granthi and jalandhara bandha with Rudra granthi. Granthis prevents the flow of prana and sushumna nadi and inhibits the flow of our chakras and Kundalini Shakti.

Brahma granthi is the first knot linked to Mooladhara and Swadhistana chakra. These are connected to our survival instincts and desires. When you get past the Brahma granthi, Kundalini energy receives an opportunity to wander up and past the Mooladhara and Swadhistana chakra without being drawn back by the instinctive traits of our personality.

The second knot is Vishnu granthi. It is linked to Manipura and Anahata chakra. These two chakras are connected to our emotional and mental sides. Manipura chakra controls our energy body (pranamaya kosha) and affects digestion and metabolism. Anahata controls our mental body (manomaya kosha). Together, the two affect our physical body – annamaya kosha. To transcend Vishnu granthi is no longer bound to physical, mental, and emotional desires. Relationships and energies take on a different character and meaning and are no longer limited to one's wants and needs.

The last knot is Rudra granthi, linked to Vishuddhi and Ajna chakra. Vishuddhi and Ajna control our body of intuition (vijnamaya kosha). When you get past the Rudra granthi, identifying with the ego stops. The experience of unmanifested consciousness appears in the Ajna and Sahasrara chakras.

"Do not search, do not seek,
do not strike,
do not demand - relax.
If you relax, it will come; if
you relax, you are there.
If you relax, you start vibra-
ting with it."

SHATKARMAS

In the old Upanishads, you can read about Hatha yoga and how it is built up of shatkarmas – purification techniques. Shat means six and karma action. Shatkarmas consists of six different purification techniques. The purpose of Hatha yoga and shatkarmas is to create a balance between ida and pingala nadi, our two most crucial prana in the body, and thus also a balance and purity both physically and mentally.

Shatkarmas are also used to balance the three doshas: vata, pitta, and kapha. According to both Hatha yoga and Ayurveda, an imbalance in the doshas causes illness. The techniques are also used before pranayamas and other more advanced yoga techniques to cleanse the body of toxins and to promote a safe and successful development purely spiritually.

Refrain from attempting to learn the techniques from a book. Seek instructions from a competent teacher who has adequate experience in the field.

Shatkarmas includes the following different techniques:

1. NETI

It is a process where you clean the nasal passages. The techniques are called jala neti and sutra neti.

2. DHAUTI

A series of purification techniques are divided into three main groups: assume dhauti (internal purification), sirshadhauti (purification of the head), and hrid dhauti (purification of the neck). These techniques cleanse the entire nutrient tract from the mouth to the rectum. There are four different techniques:

1.) Shankhaprakshalana and laghooshankhaprakshalana, which cleanse the intestines.

2.) Agnisar kriya, which activates the digestive fire.

3.) Kunjal, where one cleanses the abdomen with the help of water.

4.) Vatsara dhauti, where one cleanses the intestines with air.

3. NAULI

A method to massage and strengthen the abdominal muscles.

4. BASTI

Techniques to clean the colon.

5. KAPALBHATI

Breathing technique to clean the frontal part of the brain.

6. TRATAKA

It's a technique to develop concentration power by focusing on a point or an object. Many tantric yogis believe it is the most powerful method of obtaining siddhis (paranormal abilities).

The six shatkarmas consist of different variations of exercises. Advice and contraindications should be adhered to. Only jala neti (nasal rinsing) and trataka are recommended during pregnancy. While shatkarmas are cleansing and invigorating, they are not the primary purpose of the techniques. Shatkarmas are done to promote the health of those who practice yoga and to awaken and direct the energies in the body and mind safely so they do not flow the wrong way. People suffering from any medical illness should consult a competent teacher before exercising.

JALA NETI / NOSE RINSE

Jala neti is a purification technique all yogis practice before each yoga session. Jala neti cleanses the nasal passages and sinuses from mucus and contaminants. The air can then flow freely through the nose. It counteracts respiratory tract illnesses and promotes healthy ears, eyes, and throat. Tensions in the face are released. It has a calming effect on the brain. Anxiety, anger, and depression are relieved. Jala neti stimulates nerve endings in the nose and promotes the sense of smell. A balance is created between the right and left nostrils and the right and left sides of the brain; it, in turn, creates a balance and harmony between the body and the mind. The most important thing is that jala neti helps awaken Ajna chakra.

"Who am I?
Am I my body, or can
I experience it?
Am I my thoughts, or do
I hear them?
Am I my feelings, or do
I feel them?
Am I my intuition, or do
I sense it?
Who am I? I cannot be two?
I am the being,
the consciousness,
the one who experiences
everything.
In myself but also around
I'm that, it's me.
Om Tat Tvasi"
I'm that, it's me.
Om Tat Tvasi"

Did you like the book? Feel free to follow me on my social media, share and like, tell your friends about the books, and feel free to write an honest review; one or two lines don't matter. All support is precious. Thanks!

On my Facebook page and Instagram, I post exciting news and tips on temporary offers and benefits you can take advantage of. I often also post my yoga routine and other things related to nutrition and health that may be interesting to take part in. So feel free to join them so you don't miss anything interesting:

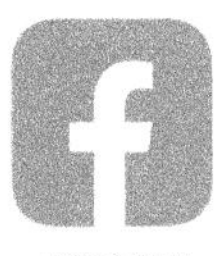 *facebook.com/bhagwanoneofakindbooks*

 *instagram.com/bhagwanoneofakindbooks/*

MY BOOKS AND BOOK SERIES

I have two book series that have different audiences. Great Yoga Books – is a series with the most comprehensive fact books on yoga for those who want to explore the subject in depth. Here, you will also find classic yoga books that are rarely translated, such as Patanjali's Yoga Sutras and Hatha Yoga Pradipika. My second series, Yoga Beyond the Poses: The Ultimate Beginner's Guide to Yoga, covers one yoga topic at a time and is extra easy to read with larger text. For those who find it challenging to read extensive books and want a good and broad overview of the subject quickly. Both series are also available as audiobooks.

★★★★★

TEACHING YOGA
&
MEDITATION
BEYOND
THE POSES

BESTSELLING AUTHOR

Shreyananda Natha

Teaching Yoga and Meditation Beyond the Poses – A unique and practical workbook!

Teaching Yoga and Meditation Beyond the Poses – A unique and practical workbook for aspiring yoga teachers who want to teach yoga and meditation beyond the poses.

Teaching Yoga and Meditation Beyond the Poses is a unique and essential resource for new and experienced teachers and a guide for all yoga students interested in refining their skills and knowledge. Teaching Yoga and Meditation is also ideal as a core textbook in yoga teacher training programs.

The book covers fundamental yoga philosophy and history topics, including a historical presentation of classical yoga literature: Yoga Sutras of Patanjali, Bhagavad Gita, etc. Each of the seven major styles of yoga is described, from Hatha yoga, Raja yoga, Tantra yoga, Bhakti yoga, and Kundalini yoga, to knowledge about the chakras, Ayurveda and magic mantras and yantras. The book provides extensive support and tools for teaching integrated and classical yoga (asanas), breathing techniques (pranayama), deep relaxation (Yoga Nidra), and meditation (Ajapa Japa). The book is divided into eight modules with associated knowledge tests and com-plete yoga and meditation classes.

https://rb.gy/9s6edj

Download the ***AUDIOBOOK*** *here!*
SCAN QR-CODE or go to:
https://bit.ly/4605zNW

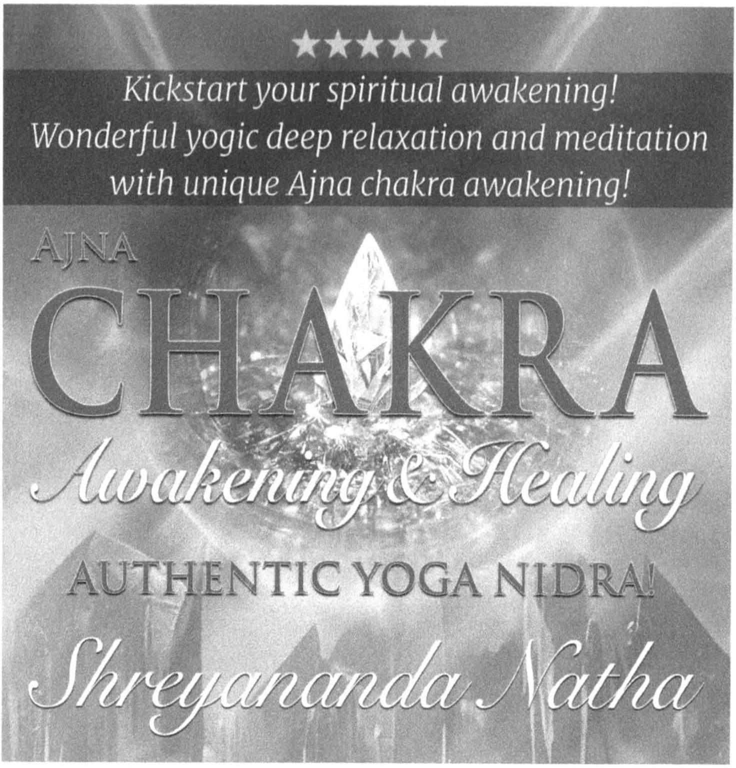